COMPLETE GUIDE TO UNDERSTANDING WRIST ARTHROPLASTY

Expert Insights On Surgical Techniques, Recovery, And Long-Term Outcomes For Optimal Joint Replacement

KLEIN HOYLE

Disclaimer

The content in this book is based on the author's expertise and comprehension of the topic. The author has no affiliation or link with any corporation, business, or person. This book is meant to give general information and educational material only, and it should not be interpreted as professional medical advice. Always seek the advice of a skilled healthcare expert if you have any queries about medical issues or treatments. The author and publisher expressly disclaim any responsibility resulting directly or indirectly from the use or use of the information included in this book.

Table of Contents

ABOUT THIS BOOK

The "Complete Guide to Understanding Wrist Arthroplasty" is an invaluable resource for both experienced orthopedic surgeons and those new to the profession, providing a thorough examination of a surgical treatment critical in restoring wrist function and relieving pain. This book guides readers through the complex environment of wrist arthroplasty with great attention to detail, beginning with an educational introduction in Chapter 1. Readers will learn about the history and progress of wrist arthroplasty, as well as the most prevalent diseases that need this procedure and a complete grasp of wrist anatomy as it relates to surgical intervention.

Moving effortlessly into Chapter 2, the emphasis changes to patient assessment and preoperative planning. This section provides surgeons with the information they need to traverse the difficulties of patient selection and preparation, from identifying eligible candidates to explaining the diagnostic testing and imaging methods required for informed decision-making. Chapter 3 goes into surgical methods and approaches, offering a thorough review of possible procedures, surgical approaches, and the complexities of anesthetic management.

Chapter 4 focuses on implant selection and prosthetic design, providing a thorough study of the different implant types, selection variables, and the most recent developments driving prosthesis design. Chapter 5 walks readers through the complexities of intraoperative concerns, from surgical procedures to dealing with unanticipated difficulties, ensuring physicians are well-prepared to handle the operating theater with confidence.

Chapter 6 focuses on postoperative care and rehabilitation, stressing the importance of immediate and long-term patient treatment in achieving optimal results. This part provides a road map for complete patient care, including everything from rehabilitation regimens to postoperative complications treatment.

Chapter 7 delves into functional outcomes and expectations, offering insight into expected improvements after surgery, variables impacting results, and appropriate patient expectations. Meanwhile, Chapter 8 covers the inevitable obstacles, looking at probable consequences and preventative tactics, as well as reasons and procedures for revision surgery.

Chapter 9 delves into the special concerns and controversies surrounding wrist arthroplasty, offering insight into its applicability across varied patient demographics as well as the ethical and legal issues that arise in this sector. Finally, Chapter 10 looks to the future, covering current research trends, predicted technology developments, and prospects for cooperation and innovation.

In conclusion, the "Complete Guide to Understanding Wrist Arthroplasty" is an authoritative compendium that provides vital insights and practical assistance that transcend traditional limits, confirming its position as an indispensable resource in the arsenal of orthopedic surgeons worldwide.

CHAPTER 1

Introduction To Wrist Arthroplasty

What Is Wrist Arthroplasty?

Wrist arthroplasty, commonly known as wrist joint replacement, is a surgical treatment used to restore function and relieve discomfort in the wrist joint by replacing damaged or diseased portions with artificial components. This technique is usually considered when more conservative therapies, such as medicines and physical therapy, have failed to offer sufficient relief. Arthroplasty improves the patient's quality of life and restores mobility by mimicking the natural movement and function of the wrist joint.

History And Development Of Wrist Arthroplasty

The history of wrist arthroplasty may be traced back to the early twentieth century when the first efforts focused on simple joint fusions to treat severe arthritis. However, these operations often resulted in reduced wrist movement and function. Materials, surgical methods, and implant design have advanced throughout time, resulting in more complex wrist arthroplasty treatments.

The first generation of wrist arthroplasty implants appeared in the 1970s, with a focus on rheumatoid arthritis treatment. These early implants encountered issues such as implant loosening and limited durability. Subsequent generations of implants addressed these shortcomings by using superior materials like titanium and ceramic, as well as more sophisticated designs that better imitated normal wrist anatomy and function.

Wrist arthroplasty is still evolving, with continual research and innovation aiming at increasing implant lifetime, refining surgical procedures, and broadening surgical indications. Modern wrist arthroplasty treatments provide patients with better results and a wider range of motion than previous approaches.

Common Conditions Causing Wrist Arthroplasty

Wrist arthroplasty may be advised for a variety of disorders resulting in wrist discomfort, stiffness, and loss of function. Wrist arthroplasty is often performed for the following conditions:

1. **Osteoarthritis:** This degenerative joint condition is characterized by cartilage degradation in the wrist joint, which causes pain, edema, and stiffness.

2. Rheumatoid arthritis is an inflammatory disease that causes inflammation of the synovial membrane, resulting in discomfort, deformity, and joint damage.

3. Post-Traumatic Arthritis: Arthritis is caused by a traumatic injury to the wrist, such as fractures or ligament tears, resulting in joint instability and degeneration.

4. Kienböck's Disease is an uncommon disorder characterized by avascular necrosis (loss of blood flow) of the lunate bone in the wrist, which causes discomfort and restricted mobility.

5. Carpal collapse is the progressive collapse of the carpal bones owing to a variety of conditions, resulting in wrist instability and dysfunction.

Overview Of Wrist Anatomy Relevant For Arthroplasty

Understanding the anatomy of the wrist is critical to completing effective arthroplasty surgeries. The wrist joint is a complicated system made up of many bones, ligaments, tendons, and cartilage that all work together to produce stability and motion.

Wrist arthroplasty mostly involves the radius, ulna, and carpal bones (including the scaphoid, lunate, triquetrum, and pisiform).

The wrist joint is a condyloid joint, which allows for flexion, extension, abduction, adduction, and circumduction motions. Ligaments that surround the wrist joint offer stability and limit excessive mobility. The articular surfaces of the wrist bones are lined with smooth cartilage, allowing for frictionless movement.

Wrist arthroplasty involves replacing damaged or diseased portions of the wrist joint with prosthetic components composed of metal, plastic, or ceramic materials. These components are intended to recreate the normal structure and function of the wrist joint, restoring stability, relieving discomfort, and increasing the range of motion for the patient.

CHAPTER 2

Patient Evaluation And Preoperative Preparation

Evaluating Candidates For Wrist Arthroplasty

Before delving into the complex realm of wrist arthroplasty, it is critical to determine who is an appropriate candidate for this treatment. Not everyone who has wrist discomfort or dysfunction can benefit from arthroplasty. Patient evaluation is a detailed examination of many criteria, including medical history, symptoms, past therapies, and the severity of the problem.

First and foremost, knowing the patient's medical history is critical. Conditions including arthritis, trauma, and congenital abnormalities may have a substantial influence on decision-making.

Patients with severe arthritis, especially rheumatoid arthritis or osteoarthritis, may benefit from wrist arthroplasty.

Next, evaluate the patient's symptoms. Persistent discomfort, stiffness, edema, and a restricted range of motion are all signs that wrist arthroplasty might be advantageous. However, it is critical to distinguish between symptoms produced by wrist arthritis and those caused by other diseases.

Candidates are also evaluated based on previous treatments. Patients who have exhausted conservative treatment options such as medicine, physical therapy, or corticosteroid injections may be candidates for arthroplasty. Furthermore, knowing the patient's expectations and objectives for the surgery is critical in assessing eligibility.

Diagnostic Testing And Imaging Techniques

When a patient is identified as a candidate for wrist arthroplasty, diagnostic testing, and imaging methods are used to confirm the diagnosis and determine the severity of the problem. These tools give essential insights into the anatomy and pathophysiology of the wrist joint, which helps with treatment planning and surgical decisions.

X-rays are often the first line of imaging utilized to assess the wrist joint. They may show symptoms of arthritis, joint space constriction, bone spurs, and abnormalities. Magnetic Resonance Imaging (MRI) may be used to evaluate soft tissue components including ligaments, tendons, and cartilage, giving a complete picture of the joint's health.

In certain circumstances, Computed Tomography (CT) scans may be used to generate comprehensive three-dimensional pictures of the wrist joint, especially in complicated cases or when determining bone quality for implant placement. In addition, ultrasonography may be used to assess soft tissue structures and discover anomalies.

Diagnostic testing, such as blood tests, may also be conducted to look for inflammatory markers, autoimmune illnesses, or metabolic abnormalities that might affect surgical outcomes or suggest underlying systemic problems.

Preparing Patients For Surgery

Preoperative planning is critical for the success of wrist arthroplasty and improving patient outcomes. This phase requires a coordinated effort from the surgical team, the patient, and other healthcare providers to resolve any medical, psychological, or logistical issues.

First and foremost, patients get a thorough preoperative evaluation to determine their general health and identify any possible hazards or contraindications to surgery. This evaluation may involve a physical examination, a review of your medical history, laboratory testing, and, if required, clearance from additional doctors.

Patients are also informed about the process, including what to anticipate before, during, and after surgery. This includes information regarding anesthetic alternatives, possible risks and problems, the expected recovery time, and postoperative rehabilitation.

Understanding Risks And Benefits

Wrist arthroplasty, like any other surgical treatment, has risks and advantages that must be thoroughly weighed before starting. Understanding the risks and benefits is critical for patients to make educated treatment choices.

The major advantage of wrist arthroplasty is pain alleviation and increased function, which allows patients to restore mobility and resume everyday activities with less discomfort. Arthroplasty, which replaces damaged or diseased joint surfaces with prosthetic components, may restore stability and joint mobility.

However, it is important to understand that no surgical operation is without danger. Wrist arthroplasty problems may include infection, implant loosening or failure, nerve or blood vessel damage, stiffness, and persistent discomfort. Patients must assess the possible dangers and advantages and address any concerns with their healthcare professional.

Furthermore, the long-term success of wrist arthroplasty is determined by many variables, including patient selection, surgical technique, implant design, and postoperative care. Understanding the risks and advantages of the surgery allows patients to make educated choices and actively engage in their treatment plans.

CHAPTER 3

Surgical Techniques And Approaches

Overview Of Different Wrist Arthroplasty Procedures

Wrist arthroplasty is a surgical technique used to relieve pain and restore function in people suffering from wrist arthritis or other wrist-related diseases. There are many distinct techniques available in the field of wrist arthroplasty, each with its own set of benefits and disadvantages.

Total wrist arthroplasty (TWA) involves replacing the entire joint with an artificial implant. This operation is normally reserved for patients with severe wrist arthritis who have not responded to other conservative therapies.

Another form is partial wrist arthroplasty, which involves replacing just a section of the joint with an implant. This might be useful for those with less severe arthritis or a particular joint injury.

Wrist arthroplasty uses a variety of implants, including those composed of metal, ceramic, or a mix of materials. The choice of implant is determined by the patient's anatomy, the level of joint injury, and the surgeon's preferences.

Comparison Of Surgical Approaches

During wrist arthroplasty, surgeons have various options for accessing the joint. Each strategy has benefits and disadvantages, and the approach chosen is determined by criteria such as the patient's anatomy, the exact treatment being done, and the surgeon's expertise.

One typical way is the dorsal approach, which allows the surgeon to reach the wrist joint from the back of the hand.

This method gives excellent exposure to the joint and is often utilized for surgeries like complete wrist arthroplasty.

Another option is the volar approach, which allows the surgeon to reach the joint from the front of the hand. This method may be recommended for particular surgeries or people with certain anatomical needs.

In addition to these fundamental techniques, surgeons may use variants and adaptations depending on the particular patient and the specific aims of the operation.

Anesthesia Options For Wrist Arthroplasty

Wrist arthroplasty may be done under a variety of anesthetic options, based on the patient's preferences, medical history, and the surgeon's recommendations.

Local, regional, and general anesthesia are some of the most common methods.

Local anesthetic includes injecting drugs into the wrist to numb it. This permits the patient to be awake during the surgery while avoiding discomfort.

Regional anesthesia, such as a nerve block, numbs a wider portion of the arm and hand. This may give more complete pain relief and may be chosen for longer or more complicated procedures.

General anesthesia causes unconsciousness, enabling the patient to be oblivious and pain-free during the treatment. This option is often reserved for individuals who cannot handle other types of anesthesia or for procedures requiring a higher degree of sedation.

The choice of anesthesia is determined by criteria such as the patient's general health, the difficulty of the operation, and the surgeon's preferences.

Surgical Instruments And Equipment

Wrist arthroplasty needs specific devices and equipment to be performed safely and properly. These might include surgical tools like scalpels, retractors, and drills, as well as imaging equipment like X-ray machines or fluoroscopy devices.

Surgeons may also employ customized implants developed expressly for wrist arthroplasty, such as prosthetic components comprised of metal, ceramic, or other materials.

The precise surgery being done, the surgeon's expertise and preferences, and the availability of technology and resources in the operating room all influence the selection of tools and equipment used. A successful operation requires that all relevant tools and equipment be properly disinfected and prepped.

Chapter 4:

Implant Selection And Prosthetic Design

There Are Many Kinds Of Wrist Implants Available

Wrist arthroplasty, often known as wrist replacement surgery, includes a variety of implants, each intended to address specific diseases and patient demands. One popular form is the whole wrist implant, which replaces both the radial and ulnar sides of the wrist joint. Another form is the partial wrist implant, which replaces just one side of the joint, such as the radial or ulnar side.

Total wrist implants are often made of metal components that articulate with one another, simulating the natural movement of the wrist joint. These components are often composed of materials like titanium or cobalt-chromium alloys, which are both robust and biocompatible. To ensure stability and smooth movement, partial wrist implants may also include plastic or ceramic components.

In addition to complete and partial implants, there are customized implants for particular disorders such as rheumatoid arthritis and post-traumatic arthritis. These implants may have unique characteristics to meet the patient's specific anatomy and biomechanics.

Factors Influencing Implant Selection

The kind of implant used for wrist arthroplasty is determined by various criteria, including the patient's age, activity level, medical history, and severity of their wrist issue. Younger, more active individuals may benefit from implants with increased durability and range of motion, while elderly patients or those with significant health conditions may need implants with a focus on stability and lifespan.

Another essential factor is the patient's bone quality and architecture. Some implants may need more bone excision or alteration than others, therefore surgeons must thoroughly examine each patient's anatomy to select the best implant choice.

Furthermore, the surgeon's expertise and knowledge of various implant systems may impact the implant selection. Surgeons may have preferences depending on their training, experience, and prior success with certain implant designs.

Understanding Prosthetic Design

Prosthesis design is crucial to the success of wrist arthroplasty surgery. The objective of prosthesis design is to closely mimic the natural anatomy and biomechanics of the wrist joint while maintaining stability and longevity.

Prosthesis design considerations include the form and size of implant components, materials employed, and articulating surfaces that allow for smooth movement. Implants may be made to resemble the form of the native wrist bones, with characteristics like concave or convex surfaces to aid with optimal alignment and function.

Furthermore, new prosthesis designs often use innovative materials and manufacturing processes to improve performance and lifespan. To stimulate bone ingrowth and increase implant durability, certain implants may include porous coatings or 3D-printed components.

Latest Innovations In Wrist Arthroplasty Implants

Recent technological and surgical advancements have resulted in various advances in wrist arthroplasty implants. One major advance is the creation of modular implant systems, which enable surgeons to tailor implant components to the patient's specific anatomy and pathology.

Another new trend is the use of patient-specific implants that are developed using preoperative imaging scans of the patient's wrist. These bespoke implants may give a more exact fit and alignment, possibly increasing results while lowering the risk of problems.

Furthermore, researchers are looking at new materials and surface treatments to increase the function and lifetime of wrist implants. For example, implant surfaces may be coated with chemicals that minimize friction and wear, hence preventing implant loosening and failure over time.

Overall, continuous research and development activities are driving innovation in wrist arthroplasty implants, to improve patient outcomes and extend treatment choices for those with severe wrist disorders.

CHAPTER 5

Intraoperative Considerations

A Step-By-Step Guide To Wrist Arthroplasty Surgery

When it comes to wrist arthroplasty surgery, precision is vital for a positive result. Here's a thorough explanation of the procedure:

1. Preparation: Before beginning surgery, the patient is properly positioned on the operating table, often lying on their back with their arm extended and supported. The surgical team prepares the operative site by cleaning and sterilizing it.

2. Anesthesia is used to keep the patient comfortable and pain-free during the treatment. Depending on the patient's health and the surgeon's discretion, a general or regional anesthetic may be used.

3. Incision: The surgeon creates an incision above the wrist joint using the predefined surgical method. This might be a posterior or anterior approach, depending on the patient's anatomy and the unique needs of the treatment.

4. Exposure: After making the incision, the surgeon gently cuts through the layers of tissue to expose the wrist joint. Specialized retractors may be utilized during surgery to provide optimum exposure and visibility.

5. Joint Access: With the joint accessible, the surgeon may examine the injured or diseased areas of the wrist joint. This may include removing diseased cartilage or bone pieces and prepping the joint surfaces for the arthroplasty implant.

6. Implant Placement: The selected wrist arthroplasty implant is carefully put into the joint area to ensure good alignment and fit. The surgeon may use specialized devices to precisely and firmly install the implant into the joint.

7. **Closure:** After the implant is in place and the joint stability has been established, the surgeon closes the incision with sutures or surgical staples. The incision is subsequently treated, and a splint or cast may be used to support the wrist during the early stages of recovery.

8. **Postoperative Care:** Following surgery, the patient is constantly observed in the recovery room to facilitate a seamless transition from anesthesia. Pain management and rehabilitation techniques are used to help with healing and promote optimum joint function.

Managing Intraoperative Complications

Several intraoperative problems may occur during wrist arthroplasty surgery, necessitating timely detection and care to guarantee a successful result. Common complications include:

1. **Nerve Injury:** Damage to adjacent nerves during surgical dissection might cause sensory or motor impairments in the hand and wrist. To prevent nerve injury, the surgeon must use care and accuracy; if nerve damage occurs, immediate surgery may be necessary.

2. **Vascular Injury:** Inadvertent injury to blood vessels supplying the hand and wrist may cause bleeding and reduced blood flow. Electrocautery and ligation are two hemostasis methods that may be used to reduce bleeding and restore vascular integrity.

3. **Implant Malposition:** Improper placement or alignment of the arthroplasty implant may impair joint function and stability. Real-time imaging, intraoperative evaluation, and rigorous surgical techniques are required to ensure proper implant placement.

4. **Infection:** Surgical site infection is a major issue during wrist arthroplasty surgery, demanding rigorous

sterile methods and perioperative antimicrobial treatment. Prompt detection and control of infection are critical for avoiding complications and promoting favorable results.

5. Implant Failure: Even with precise surgical technique, implant failure may occur owing to implant loosening, dislocation, or wear. Close follow-up and monitoring are required to assess implant stability and performance over time, with revision surgery an option if necessary.

Surgical Tips And Techniques

Successful wrist arthroplasty surgery requires a mix of technical competence, surgical knowledge, and meticulous attention to detail. Here are some useful suggestions and approaches for attaining the best results:

1. Anatomical grasp: A detailed grasp of wrist anatomy is required for proper surgical planning and execution.

Learn about the complicated architecture and biomechanics of the wrist joint so that you can traverse the surgical anatomy with accuracy.

2. **Patient Selection:** Careful patient selection is required to identify eligible candidates for wrist arthroplasty surgery. When determining surgical candidacy, consider age, activity level, comorbidities, and joint pathology.

3. **Surgical Approach:** Determine the best surgical approach based on the patient's anatomy, the location of the disease, and the surgeon's experience and skill. Both posterior and anterior techniques have benefits and drawbacks, so choose the strategy that best fits the particular patient and surgical objectives.

4. **Implant Selection:** Choosing the proper implant is critical to obtaining peak joint function and lifetime. When deciding on the best implant choice, consider the implant's design, material composition, size, and compatibility with the patient's anatomy.

5. Intraoperative Imaging: Use imaging modalities like fluoroscopy or intraoperative ultrasonography to help in implant placement and alignment. Real-time visualization may assist assure precise implant location and improve joint biomechanics.

Posterior And Anterior Surgical Approaches

Wrist arthroplasty surgery may be done utilizing either a posterior or anterior surgical technique, each of which provides significant benefits and considerations.

The posterior approach:

• Allows direct access to the wrist joint and extensor tendons.

• Provides great exposure of the distal radius and carpal bones.

• Improves implant placement and fixation in the radial and ulnar columns.

• May increase risk of extensor tendon damage and scar formation.

Anterior Approach:

• Provides immediate access to wrist joints and flexor tendons.

• Preserves dorsal wrist function while minimizing extensor tendon disruption.

• Ensures clear sight of the carpal bones and proximal row.

• Technical challenges may arise with severe deformities or limited exposure.

The pathology's location, surgeon preference, and patient-specific variables all influence the surgical method used. Both procedures have shown success in the treatment of wrist arthritis and may provide positive results when done by skilled surgeons using proper patient selection and surgical technique.

CHAPTER 6

Post-Operative Care And Rehabilitation

Immediate Postoperative Care At The Hospital

Following a wrist arthroplasty, urgent postoperative care in the hospital is critical for a smooth recovery and excellent results. Patients are often intensively observed in the recovery room or critical care unit shortly after the operation. During this period, healthcare experts will check vital signs, manage pain, and look for symptoms of problems like infection or excessive bleeding.

Pain management is a vital part of postoperative treatment. Patients may be given pain medication intravenously or orally to assist relieve their agony. Additionally, elevating the injured wrist might help minimize swelling and discomfort. Ice packs may also be used occasionally to reduce swelling and pain.

Furthermore, patients should begin mild range of motion exercises as soon as feasible after surgery. These exercises assist in reducing stiffness and improve recovery. However, to prevent damaging the surgical site, it is essential to follow the surgeon's exact recommendations for the time and intensity of these workouts.

In certain situations, patients may need a splint or cast to immobilize their wrists during the early phases of healing. This protects the surgery site and promotes healthy recovery. The healthcare provider will explain how to care for the splint or cast and when it may be safely removed.

Close communication among the patient, healthcare personnel, and family members is critical during the initial postoperative period. Any concerns or changes in symptoms should be addressed to your healthcare practitioner right away to provide proper treatment and assistance during this vital stage of recovery.

Rehabilitation Protocol After Wrist Arthroplasty

Following wrist arthroplasty, a coordinated rehabilitation plan is required to improve outcomes and restore function. The rehabilitation routine will normally begin soon after surgery and last several weeks to months, depending on the patient's progress and surgical method.

In the early phases of rehabilitation, the emphasis is on a mild range of motion exercises and strengthening activities. Physical therapists will collaborate with patients to create a customized fitness program based on their unique requirements and objectives. Wrist flexion and extension, forearm rotation, and grip strength exercises are some of the possible workouts.

As the patient's rehabilitation improves, more sophisticated exercises may be offered to enhance strength, flexibility, and function. These may involve proprioceptive training, which improves coordination and balance, as well as functional exercises that mimic real-life motions and tasks.

In addition to planned exercise regimens, rehabilitation after wrist arthroplasty may include manual therapy, ultrasound, or electrical stimulation to alleviate pain and inflammation and improve tissue recovery.

Throughout the rehabilitation process, progress must be closely monitored to ensure that the program is successful and that modifications may be made as necessary. The objective of rehabilitation after wrist arthroplasty is to assist patients in restoring optimum function and resume everyday activities as soon and safely as feasible.

Common Postoperative Complications And Management

While wrist arthroplasty is often a safe and successful treatment, problems might arise in certain circumstances. Common postoperative consequences include infection, implant loosening or failure, nerve damage, and joint stiffness or instability.

Infection is a significant consequence that needs immediate antibiotic treatment and, in rare situations, surgical removal of diseased tissue or implants. Implant loosening or failure may need revision surgery to replace the compromised components and restore functionality.

Nerve damage may occur during surgery, causing temporary or permanent loss of feeling or motor function in the hand or wrist. Physical therapy and rehabilitation may reduce the severity of nerve damage and facilitate healing.

Another possible consequence after wrist arthroplasty is joint stiffness or instability. Physical therapy and rehabilitation are critical for restoring range of motion, strength, and stability to the joints. In certain circumstances, further surgical treatments may be required to treat chronic stiffness or instability.

Early detection and treatment of problems is critical for reducing their influence on outcomes and maximizing patient recovery after wrist arthroplasty.

Long-Term Follow-Up And Monitoring

Long-term follow-up and monitoring are critical components of therapy after wrist arthroplasty to guarantee the best possible results and discover any potential issues early. Patients often have follow-up meetings with their surgeon at regular intervals after surgery.

During these follow-up sessions, the surgeon will evaluate the patient's progress, watch for symptoms of problems, and make any required changes to the treatment plan. Additional imaging examinations, including X-rays or MRI scans, may be performed to assess the implant's and surrounding tissues' integrity.

In addition to scheduled follow-up consultations with the surgeon, patients may continue to work with physical therapists or other rehabilitation specialists to maintain and enhance wrist and hand strength, flexibility, and function.

Long-term surveillance after wrist arthroplasty is critical for spotting any issues early and responding quickly to avoid additional injury or deterioration. With proper follow-up and monitoring, most patients may anticipate seeing considerable improvements in pain and function after wrist arthroplasty, as well as long-term success with their implant.

CHAPTER 7

Functional Outcomes And Expectations

Expected Functional Improvement Following Wrist Arthroplasty

Wrist arthroplasty has the potential to significantly enhance functional outcomes for people suffering from wrist arthritis and other severe disorders. The major purpose of this operation is to restore mobility, strength, and stability to the wrist joint, which will improve general hand and wrist function.

Patients who undergo wrist arthroplasty should anticipate seeing significant improvements in their functional skills. These may include better range of motion, pain relief, improved grip strength, and wrist joint stability. The particular degree of improvement varies based on the patient's pre-existing condition, the kind of arthroplasty done, and the surgical intervention's success rate.

One of the most noticeable benefits patients often report is a dramatic decrease in discomfort. Wrist arthroplasty, which replaces damaged or deteriorating joint surfaces with prosthetic components, may relieve arthritis or other degenerative disorders' discomfort. This alleviation allows sufferers to accomplish their everyday tasks more comfortably and easily.

Furthermore, wrist arthroplasty may improve the range of motion, enabling patients to move their wrists more freely and participate in activities that were previously difficult or impossible. This enhanced flexibility may have a significant influence on a person's quality of life by allowing them to execute jobs like typing, writing, cooking, and driving more easily and efficiently.

Furthermore, effective wrist arthroplasty often results in enhanced grip strength. Patients often report that by restoring wrist joint stability and correcting underlying structural abnormalities, they can hold items more securely and do manual activities with more confidence and accuracy. Individuals who depend on their hands for a job or enjoyment may benefit the most from this increase in grip strength.

In conclusion, patients who have wrist arthroplasty should expect a variety of functional benefits, including less discomfort, better range of motion, increased grip strength, and improved overall hand and wrist function. These enhancements may have a significant impact on patients' everyday lives, allowing them to recover independence, productivity, and pleasure from things that they may have previously struggled with.

Factors Affecting Functional Outcome

While wrist arthroplasty may provide considerable functional improvement for many patients, the final result can be impacted by several variables. Understanding these characteristics may help patients and healthcare professionals establish reasonable expectations and increase the likelihood of a good result.

One of the most important elements influencing functional results is the patient's general health and medical history. Patients with pre-existing diseases such as diabetes, obesity, or cardiovascular disease may be more likely to have problems and a delayed recovery after wrist arthroplasty. Similarly, individuals with a history of smoking or drug misuse may have slower recovery and inferior functional results.

The degree and type of the underlying wrist problem have a significant impact on functional results. Patients with severe arthritis or substantial joint degeneration may see less functional improvement than those with milder or less advanced diseases. Furthermore, individuals with complicated wrist abnormalities or instability may need additional surgical treatments or rehabilitation to attain the best functional results.

The kind of arthroplasty technique used may also affect functional results. Different surgical procedures and prosthetic designs may result in varied levels of functional improvement and long-term durability. Implant selection, surgical strategy, and postoperative rehabilitation regimens all influence the procedure's success and the patient's functional recovery.

Furthermore, patient compliance with surgical rehabilitation and follow-up treatment has a considerable impact on functional results. Adherence to recommended exercises, activity limitations, and medication regimes is critical for encouraging healing, reducing problems, and increasing functional recovery. Patients who actively engage in their treatment and adhere to medical recommendations are more likely to have good functional results after wrist arthroplasty.

In conclusion, various variables may impact the functional results of wrist arthroplasty, including the patient's general health, the severity of the underlying illness, the kind of treatment used, and the patient's compliance with postsurgical care. Patients may establish reasonable expectations and improve their chances of success by taking these aspects into account and working together with their healthcare professionals.

Realistic Expectations For Patients

Setting reasonable expectations is critical for individuals having wrist arthroplasty so that they may get a favorable result without disappointment. While this operation may result in considerable functional improvement for many people, it is important to note that the outcomes may differ from patient to patient.

First and foremost, patients should recognize that wrist arthroplasty is not a panacea and may not alleviate all symptoms or limits. While the operation seeks to enhance wrist function and minimize discomfort, the joint may not be fully restored to its pre-injury or pre-arthritis form. Some residual discomfort or functional restrictions may remain, particularly in individuals with severe or complicated wrist disorders.

Furthermore, patients should be informed that the recovery period after wrist arthroplasty may be protracted and requires patience and dedication. While some people see immediate improvements in function and comfort, others may need many months of therapy and progressive strengthening to attain the best results. It is critical to closely follow postoperative instructions, attend follow-up visits, and speak honestly with healthcare personnel about any concerns or difficulties throughout the healing process.

Furthermore, patients should realize that the outcome of wrist arthroplasty is dependent on several circumstances, including their general health, the severity of the underlying ailment, and their adherence to postoperative treatment. While healthcare experts try to improve surgical methods and prosthetic designs, all surgical procedures have inherent risks and uncertainty. Patients should carefully consider these variables and have reasonable expectations about the possible advantages and limits of wrist arthroplasty.

Overall, patients having wrist arthroplasty should approach the treatment with cautious hope and a willingness to actively participate in their care. Patients may enhance their chances of success and quality of life after surgery by establishing realistic expectations, communicating openly with healthcare staff, and sticking to postoperative guidelines.

Return To Activities And Work After Surgery

Returning to hobbies and jobs following wrist arthroplasty is a crucial milestone in patients' rehabilitation. While the timing for returning to certain activities may vary based on individual circumstances, there are some basic rules and factors to keep in mind throughout the postoperative period.

Patients should anticipate spending the first several weeks after surgery focusing on rest, wound care, and rehabilitation activities to improve healing and avoid problems. Physical therapy may be recommended to enhance the range of motion, strength, and coordination of the wrist and hands. To prevent overexertion or reinjury, follow the advice of your healthcare professional and gradually raise your activity levels as tolerated.

As recovery proceeds and functional capacities improve, patients may gradually resume activities of daily life such as dressing, grooming, and light housework. It is important to pace oneself and listen to the body's cues to avoid overdoing it and suffering setbacks in the healing process.

Returning to work following wrist arthroplasty may need extra planning, depending on the nature of the employment and the physical demands involved. Patients with sedentary desk occupations may be able to return to work sooner than those with physical tasks or heavy-lifting responsibilities. It is critical to speak with employers about any required adjustments or changes to tasks throughout the transition back to work.

Patients should also be aware of ergonomic concepts and good body mechanics to reduce stress on the wrist joint and avoid re-injury. To decrease wrist and hand strain, consider employing assistive devices, changing workstations, and adopting proper posture and lifting methods.

In summary, returning to activities and employment following wrist arthroplasty requires patience, effort, and strict adherence to postoperative instructions. Patients may effectively manage the rehabilitation process by gradually resuming activities, listening to their bodies' signals, and talking with healthcare professionals and employers.

CHAPTER 8

Complications And Revision Surgery

Overview Of Potential Complications After Wrist Arthroplasty

Wrist arthroplasty, although providing great advantages for restoring wrist function, is not without risks. Understanding these problems allows both patients and doctors to make educated choices and control expectations.

One typical problem is implant loosening. This happens when the prosthetic joint doesn't adequately merge with the surrounding bone, causing instability and pain. Infection is another major worry, as with any surgical surgery. In certain situations, patients may also suffer nerve injury, which causes numbness or paralysis in the hand and wrist.

Furthermore, there is a danger of implant wear and tear over time, which may need revision surgery. Other concerns include stiffness, instability, and ongoing discomfort after the surgery. Each patient's circumstance is unique, and the risk of problems varies depending on variables such as general health, surgical method, and implant type.

Techniques For Preventing Complications

Complications are usually better avoided than treated. Surgeons use a variety of methods to reduce the likelihood of bad outcomes during wrist arthroplasty. A thorough preoperative screening is required to detect any underlying disorders that might raise the risk of problems. Optimizing the patient's general health before surgery may also help improve results.

During the treatment, precision surgical skill is required to achieve correct implant placement and stability.

Careful soft tissue treatment reduces the danger of infection and nerve injury. Postoperative rehabilitation is crucial for encouraging healing and regaining function while lowering the risk of problems like stiffness.

Regular follow-up visits enable surgeons to carefully evaluate the patient's development and treat any issues as soon as they arise. Education is also important, as patients must grasp the significance of following surgical instructions and rehabilitation regimens to improve results and reduce the risk of complications.

Indications And Techniques Of Revision Surgery

Despite our best efforts to avoid problems, some patients may need revision surgery for a variety of reasons. Implant failure, chronic discomfort, instability, or complications such as infection or implant loosening all indicate the need for revision surgery.

The choice to conduct revision surgery is based on a thorough examination of the patient's symptoms, functional limits, and general health. Imaging examinations, such as X-rays or MRI scans, may be required to examine the status of the implant and surrounding tissues.

Revision surgery sometimes necessitates more complex operations than the first arthroplasty, since scar tissue or bone loss must be addressed. The techniques for revision surgery differ based on the individual issues and the surgeon's experience. Implant removal and replacement, bone grafting, and soft tissue repair are common techniques for treating instability or stiffness.

Case Studies In Complication Management

Case studies provide useful insights into the treatment of problems after wrist arthroplasty. Surgeons may learn from both successful and unsuccessful revisions by reviewing real-life events.

One case study may be a patient who experiences implant loosening many years after wrist arthroplasty. The surgeon may choose revision surgery to replace the loose implant with a new one and treat any underlying conditions causing the failure.

Another case study may be on a patient who gets a postoperative infection that needs extensive antibiotic therapy and perhaps implant removal. Despite the setback, the patient may still obtain an acceptable result with diligent treatment, including wound care and rehabilitation.

Each case study emphasizes the need for personalized treatment strategies and multidisciplinary teamwork among surgeons, infectious disease experts, and rehabilitation professionals in improving patient outcomes after wrist arthroplasty.

CHAPTER 9

Special Considerations And Controversies

Wrist Arthroplasty In Specific Patient Populations

Wrist arthroplasty is a flexible surgery that may be adapted to the specific demands of different patient groups, such as the elderly and sports.

Elderly people often appear with degenerative disorders such as osteoarthritis or rheumatoid arthritis, which may have a major impact on wrist function and quality of life. Wrist arthroplasty is a feasible treatment option for these patients because it replaces damaged joint surfaces with prosthetic components. However, bone quality, systemic health, and functional objectives must all be carefully considered before going with surgery.

Wrist arthroplasty in elderly patients seeks to restore mobility and relieve discomfort, enabling them to keep independence and participate in everyday activities more easily.

Athletes have special demands on their wrists owing to repeated stress and high-impact exercises. Injuries such as ligament tears, cartilage damage, or fractures may impair wrist function and performance. Wrist arthroplasty may be recommended in some circumstances if conservative therapies have failed to give enough relief or restore function. However, the choice to have surgery must balance the possible advantages with the hazards of postoperative restrictions and activity limits. Rehabilitation methods that are personalized to the athlete's unique sport and performance objectives are critical for maximizing results and reducing the risk of complications.

Controversies Around Wrist Arthroplasty

Despite its success in treating wrist diseases, wrist arthroplasty remains a source of contention among orthopedic surgeons and researchers. There are many concerns surrounding the technique, including:

Long-term Outcomes: One of the most common concerns about wrist arthroplasty is the long-term durability and function of prosthetic implants. While many patients find considerable improvements in pain relief and function immediately, concerns remain concerning implant lifespan and the potential of problems such as implant loosening or wear over time. Long-term studies are required to evaluate the durability and effectiveness of wrist arthroplasty to other therapies, such as fusion.

Patient Selection: Another point of contention is the optimal patient selection criteria for wrist arthroplasty. Some surgeons argue for expanded indications to include younger, active patients with advanced arthritis, whilst others highlight the significance of patient age, activity level, and functional expectations in assessing eligibility. Balancing the potential advantages of wrist arthroplasty with the risks of revision surgery and complications requires careful assessment of individual patient characteristics and surgical competence.

Another much-debated topic is the necessity for revision surgery after wrist arthroplasty. While contemporary implant designs are intended to reduce the likelihood of revision, problems such as implant failure, infection, or soft tissue contracture may need further surgeries. Revision surgery presents complications owing to low bone stock, changed architecture, and the possibility of worse results compared to original arthroplasty. Preventing the need for revision surgery involves thorough preoperative planning, intraoperative methods to preserve bone and soft tissue, and patient education on postoperative expectations and rehabilitation.

Alternative Treatments And Emerging Technology

In addition to wrist arthroplasty, a variety of alternative therapies and developing technologies are being investigated for the treatment of wrist disorders. This includes:

Wrist fusion, also known as arthrodesis, is a surgical procedure that immobilizes the wrist joint to reduce discomfort and stabilize it. While fusion may give long-term pain relief and functional stability, it reduces wrist mobility, which may restrict daily activities and lower quality of life. Patient selection is critical in deciding whether fusion or arthroplasty is the best treatment option.

Cartilage Restoration: New procedures for cartilage restoration attempt to protect and heal damaged joint surfaces, postponing or eliminating the need for joint replacement surgery. Autologous chondrocyte implantation (ACI), osteochondral autograft transplantation (OATS), and matrix-induced autologous chondrocyte implantation (MACI) all show promise in restoring wrist function and delaying disease progression in individuals with localized cartilage abnormalities.

3D Printing and Patient-Specific Implants: Advancements in 3D printing technology enable the creation of patient-specific implants based on individual anatomy and disease. Customized implants may enhance implant fit, stability, and lifetime, thereby improving surgical results while lowering the risk of complications. Additionally, 3D printing allows for the development of surgical guides and equipment, which aids in accurate implant placement and intraoperative navigation.

Ethical And Legal Issues With Wrist Arthroplasty

Wrist arthroplasty involves various ethical and legal issues that need serious consideration:

Informed Consent: In wrist arthroplasty, informed consent is required to ensure that patients understand the risks, benefits, and alternatives connected with the treatment. Surgeons must present patients with clear and thorough information about the expected results, possible problems, and postoperative rehabilitation regimens so that they may make educated choices regarding their treatment.

Conflicts of Interest: Orthopedic surgeons may have conflicts of interest due to industry affiliations, financial incentives, or professional prejudices that impact their treatment decisions. Maintaining openness and following ethical norms is critical to sustaining patient confidence and avoiding conflicts of interest that might jeopardize patient treatment.

Regulatory Compliance: Government bodies such as the Food and Drug Administration (FDA) regulate wrist arthroplasty implants and devices to assure their safety and effectiveness. Surgeons must follow regulatory regulations for equipment selection, off-label usage, and reporting adverse events to enhance patient safety and quality assurance.

Malpractice Liability: Orthopedic surgeons conducting wrist arthroplasty may be held accountable for malpractice if they vary from the standard of care, fail to acquire informed consent, or make surgical mistakes that cause patient injury. Maintaining competence, following evidence-based procedures, and recording patient contacts are critical measures for reducing malpractice risk and providing high-quality treatment.

CHAPTER 10

Future Directions And Advancements

Current Research Trends In Wrist Arthroplasty

In the field of wrist arthroplasty, current research efforts are always pushing the limits of what is achievable in terms of restoring function and relieving pain for patients with wrist difficulties. One major theme in current research is the refining and development of implant materials and designs. Researchers are looking at biomaterials, namely compounds that may mimic the natural qualities of bone and cartilage to improve implant durability and biocompatibility.

Furthermore, there is a strong emphasis on creating less invasive surgical procedures in wrist replacement. These procedures attempt to lessen surgical trauma, improve postoperative healing, and reduce complications. Advanced imaging technologies, such as 3D printing and virtual reality, are being used in surgical planning to enhance implant placement and alignment, resulting in better overall results.

Another exciting line of study is looking into the possibilities of regenerative medicine in wrist arthroplasty. Scientists are looking at novel ways, such as stem cell therapy and tissue engineering, to boost tissue regeneration and aid the natural healing process. These regenerative approaches have the potential to improve standard arthroplasty operations and, in certain situations, eliminate the requirement for implantation.

Predictions On Future Technological Advancements

Looking forward, the future of wrist arthroplasty seems bright, with some intriguing technical breakthroughs on the way.

Implant design and customization are one area where significant development is expected. Advances in computer-aided design (CAD) and additive manufacturing technologies are set to transform the production of patient-specific implants based on anatomical differences and disease.

Furthermore, using artificial intelligence (AI) algorithms in surgical decision-making has enormous promise for improving treatment options and predicting patient outcomes. AI-powered systems can scan large volumes of patient data to detect patterns and trends, allowing surgeons to make better judgments about surgical approach, implant selection, and post-operative care.

Furthermore, the introduction of robotic-assisted surgery is expected to change the landscape of wrist arthroplasty. Robotic platforms provide more precision, dexterity, and control during surgical operations, which may lead to better implant placement accuracy and patient outcomes.

As these technologies advance and become more widely available, they have the potential to transform the field of wrist arthroplasty.

Potential Paradigm Shifts In Wrist Arthroplasty Practice

Several possible paradigm changes in wrist arthroplasty are on the horizon, ready to alter the standard of treatment for patients with wrist disease. One such change is towards customized medicine, in which treatment procedures are adapted to each patient's specific requirements and features. Advances in genetics, imaging, and biomaterials are helping this change by allowing doctors to create personalized treatment regimens that improve patient outcomes while reducing problems.

Another paradigm change is the identification of the wrist as a biomechanically complicated joint that requires interdisciplinary care. The wrist, which was once thought to be a simple hinge joint, is now acknowledged to entail complex interactions involving bones, ligaments, tendons, and muscles. As a result, a comprehensive strategy combining orthopedic surgery, hand therapy, and rehabilitation medicine is increasingly being used to treat the multidimensional character of wrist disease.

Furthermore, there is a rising focus on patient-reported outcomes and collaborative decision-making in wrist arthroplasty therapy. Recognizing the significance of patients' preferences, objectives, and aspirations, physicians are including patients as active partners in the treatment process, allowing them to make informed decisions about their care. This patient-centered approach not only increases happiness but also promotes a collaborative therapeutic connection between patients and doctors.

Opportunities For Collaboration And Innovation In The Field

In the evolving world of wrist arthroplasty, there is significant potential for cooperation and innovation to drive development and improve patient care. Interdisciplinary cooperation among orthopedic surgeons, hand therapists, biomechanical engineers, and researchers is critical for developing innovation and synergy in treating complicated wrist diseases.

Furthermore, collaborations across academia, industry, and healthcare institutions play an important role in generating innovation and transferring research results into practice. By promoting collaborative networks and sharing resources, stakeholders may speed up the development and acceptance of innovative wrist arthroplasty technologies and treatment methods.

Furthermore, patient advocacy groups and community organizations play critical roles in increasing awareness, encouraging education, and pushing for better access to treatment for people with wrist problems. By amplifying the voices of patients and caregivers, these grassroots efforts help to shape healthcare policy and drive good change in the area of wrist arthroplasty.

Conclusion

In conclusion, understanding wrist arthroplasty is critical for both patients and healthcare practitioners. Wrist arthroplasty, as discussed throughout this thorough book, is a significant surgical alternative for those suffering from severe wrist disorders such as arthritis, trauma, or congenital anomalies who have exhausted all conservative therapy options.

Wrist arthroplasty has become a potential alternative for restoring wrist function, relieving pain, and improving overall quality of life as surgical methods and implant designs have advanced. With a variety of implant alternatives available, including total wrist arthroplasty (TWA) and partial wrist arthroplasty (PWA), surgeons may personalize the treatment strategy to each patient's particular requirements and preferences.

However, wrist arthroplasty has restrictions and possible problems. While many patients see considerable improvements after surgery, others may develop problems such as implant loosening, stiffness, or infection. As a result, cautious patient selection, complete preoperative assessment, and rigorous surgical technique are required to maximize results and reduce risks.

Furthermore, current research and innovation in wrist arthroplasty are refining surgical procedures, improving implant longevity, and expanding surgical reasons. Collaboration among doctors, academics, and industry partners is critical to advancing this emerging profession and improving long-term patient outcomes.

Beyond the technical requirements of surgery, comprehensive care for patients undergoing wrist arthroplasty is essential. This involves thorough preoperative teaching, diligent postoperative rehabilitation, and continued monitoring to track progress and handle any issues that may develop. Healthcare teams may enable patients to actively engage in their recovery journey and obtain the greatest outcomes by encouraging open communication and creating a friendly atmosphere.

In conclusion, wrist arthroplasty is an effective therapeutic choice for those suffering from severe wrist disorders, with the potential to restore function and relieve discomfort. While problems and uncertainties remain, continual advances in surgical procedures, implant design, and patient care strategies continue to improve results and broaden the scope of this discipline. By adopting a multidisciplinary approach and focusing on patient-centered care, we may improve the efficacy and safety of wrist arthroplasty for future generations.

THE END